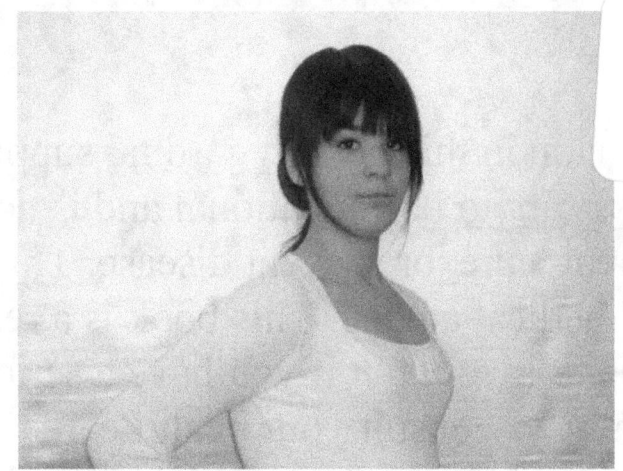

Second Edition

LUPUS CURE
OR SPONTANEOUS REMISSION

THE TRUE LIFE OF SAMANTHA GARCIA

BY
EMILIO GARCIA

DISCLAIMER

The information in this book regarding supplements and support products is meant to be educational and is not intended to diagnose, treat, cure, or prevent disease. This should not be considered medical advice. This book is a real life story that will hopefully benefit you, but if you have a serious medical condition, always consult your health-care provider. The FDA has not evaluated the products listed in this book.

What Is Lupus?

The name "lupus" comes from the Latin word for "wolf." It was used in 1700 to describe a rash across the face that looks like markings of a wolf. In the 1840s, a characteristic description of lupus by Ferdinand von Hebra of Vienna was that it was a face rash called the butterfly rash.

Can lupus run in the family? If you have a family medical history of lupus, you are thirty times more likely then someone in the general population to exhibit it. However, as is the case with most human diseases, it has environmental and genetic components as well. Seventy percent of lupus patients do not have an immediate family member with this disease.

Lupus is a disease that causes the immune system to attack the body's cells and tissues. Here one may have to redefine the concept of autoimmune diseases.

After a million years of evolution, the human immune system does not attack a normal cell. The attacks are directed at tissues in the joints, kidney, heart, brain, skin, and everywhere in the body. If the cells are not normal, then what are they? We do not know.

Some believe the immune system breaks down like an automobile. "Let us look around and see if we can find the little part that is not working and fix it." Unfortunately, humans are a little more complicated then that. We are not machines; we are a million years of bioelectrical chemistry.

"Auto" means that the body has an immune reaction against itself. Two million or more people in the United States—85 percent woman—suffer from the mysterious disease called lupus. With symptoms ranging from achy joints to kidney failure, for most people lupus is not life threatening. However, for some it *can* be life threatening.

Sir William Osler said lupus erythematosus was a systemic disorder. Then immunology, the body's responses to free radicals.

After many years, we know nothing of what lupus actually is. There is hope in the science of immunology, and the path to remission lies in allergens antigens. In traditional medicine, there is the rheumatoid factor antibodies, which may or may not cause lupus. Then there is the LE phenomenon—white cells devouring another cell.

Doctors, Food, and Health

The impact of what I am about to say may ruffle a few feathers. I must say I profoundly respect the men and woman of today's medical profession, as primitive as it may be trying to understand the parts of the human body and giving the parts names like medulla Oblongata or understanding what it controls and not have the vaguest idea of the interacting electrical biochemistry. All doctors are heroic men and woman that would like to help humanity and win the Nobel Prize. They stand against trillion-dollar corrupt food and pharmaceutical industries.

The food industries put chemicals and additives in food that cause cancer, such as diethylstibestrol to fatten livestock. The pharmaceutical industries provide prescription drugs that cause cancer and suppress the immune system. Doctors have some short-lived success cutting and drilling holes in the body and very little success with prescription drugs.

A thousand years from today, one would be in shock seeing the tools and drills that we use today to place tubes and electrical gadgets and drugs in the human body while praying things work. Shall we give up on our doctors and prescription drugs? I think not. As western society dies off from the self-inflicted epidemic of cancer and antibiotic resistant bacteria, people will find a need for good drugs, good food, and good doctors. If people live longer, they pay more for good drugs, good food, and good doctors. Sounds like Hollywood, right? However, one must remember that to live long and healthy, we must first be optimists. You want those neurochemicals from your mind talking to the receptors on the white cells in your immune system.

No one can dispute the fact that the entire human body works as interacting stimuli; neurochemicals communicate with every cell in the body. That is to say, the human body has evolved as a complicated, interacting, electrical, chemical, environmental system.

It is inept to think that disease is a self-perpetuating phenomenon. As part of the human herd (the group you live with), the mores of your culture will determine your health and what disease you will acquire. This is because of the electromagnetic fields you live in, the effect it has on your body, and the free radicals in the food your group eats.

Bad News

I woke up one morning seven years ago and found that my nine-year-old daughter had lupus. To all the doctors in the hospital this was a special event. You see, lupus rarely occurs in nine-year-old children, so they paraded us around. I was wondering what was going on.

Earlier that week, we had made a hot summer's day drive up the road to Pennsylvania to visit my sister, who lives in a small house with two kids and a dog. Samantha, my daughter, was looking out the car window. There were cows and farmhouses, and the air was clean— not like Brooklyn, where we live. Out here, there were all sorts of animals. However, in Brooklyn, there are just cats and dogs. I am just a city person; somehow I cannot get used to the life of farms and small towns with many animals and lots of trees. At night there are a million stars, though. We see very few stars in Brooklyn because of bad air and the city lights.

It was not the first time I had been to my sister's house. Everything seemed to stop—no traffic jams, no crowds in mass transit. The kids had a great time running all over town. No one seemed to worry about them. My sister even leaves her door open at night. I will never get used to it.

One day I noticed a rash on Samantha's face. I took her to the doctor, and he said she had lupus. We then took her to a specialist, who said that Samantha had, at most, five years to live. He prescribed 40mg of prednisone per day. That is a devastating dose of prednisone for a child. I had no idea what lupus or prednisone was at the time. Like most people, I went to the doctor in a time of crisis and had to learn everything on my own after the diagnosis.

It's important to understand the mental frame of reference the doctor is coming from and what he understands about the disease he is dealing with. What references is he working with, and what makes him come to this diagnosis. What treatments are there? What drugs? What are the side effects, and what drugs deal with the side effects? What are the side effects of those? What is the doctor trying to accomplish?

Seniors who are given prednisone are more likely to develop high blood pressure. In addition, my child developed high blood pressure. They can add to the research that children are likely to develop high blood pressure. Now we have two problems instead of one: lupus and high blood pressure.

Some drugs, like cytoxan and all anticoagulants, one must say no to because of the side effects. Anticoagulant therapy is extremely risky and extremely unstable because of vitamin K deficiency. This can cause serious bleeding. Hypoprthrombinemia could be the cause of major hemorrhages.

Saying no to a doctor does not make you a bad person, but be careful what you say no to. All the doctors I know—doctors of pediatric hematology oncology, doctors of pediatric nephrology and hypertension, doctors of pediatric rheumatology, and so on—are good people with your best interests in mind, honorable people that care about children. Your relationship between you and your doctor should be one of mutual cooperation between two specialists. I say two specialists because you, as a parent or patient, must understand the disease. Be involved in treatment and know how treatment is affecting you or your child. Keep in mind the ancient maxim, "Primum est non nocere" (First, do no harm).

I said yes to prednisone. However, I also wanted to work hard at keeping the dosage as low as possible. When prednisone gave my daughter high blood pressure, I said yes to enalapril in order to lower it. (As I write this, Samantha is no longer taking prednisone or enalapril. Her blood pressure is normal, and she has no inflammation or any lupus-related problems.) I said yes to plaquenil to lower the dosage of prednisone.

Plaquenil is a drug that accumulates in the body over the years. Depending on the dosage, it can, in time, cause retinal toxicity and harmful disturbances to vision due to deposits of the drug in the cornea. That disappears when the drug is stopped; however, a more serious damage to the retina can occur. It may cause total blindness, which is not reversible.

No matter what your doctor says, the research is that 200 mg every *other* day is safe—not the recommended 200 mg a day. Have the eyes checked by an ophthalmologist every three months instead of six months or one year. Again, we are talking about an accumulated drug, so there is much to be concerned about, even at low dosages.

Back to prednisone, though. Doctors use prednisone to treat lupus. Prednisone is a corticosteroid similar to the natural hormone produced by your adrenal glands. It relieves inflammation, swelling, heat, redness, and pain. In addition, it is used to treat certain types of cancer. Problems with the use of prednisone include a likeliness to develop high blood pressure, stomach irritation, vomiting, restlessness, anxiety, acne, vision problems, colds or infections that last a long time, muscle weakness, appetite loss, diarrhea, vomiting of blood, weight gain, depletion of minerals in the body (especially calcium), low blood sugar, black or tarry stool, skin rash, absent menstrual periods, easy bruising, increased hair growth, or swelling in the face, lower legs, or ankles.

Today doctors spend as much time dealing with the side

effects of drugs as they do with the disease. In Samantha's case, she had high blood pressure, absent menstrual periods, easy bruising, and swelling in her face, lower legs, and ankles. Also, depletion of calcium in her body was stunting her growth. To minimize this, one of the doctors prescribed enalapril. I say "one of her doctors" because with a disease like lupus you have many doctors. Lupus can affect different parts of the body, and each specialist will prescribe something for that particular symptom.

That is what you go to your doctor for—that miracle pill that you think is going to make everything go away. After years of mental, physical, environmental, and dietary abuse, you get sick. You go to your doctor, he gives you a pill, and all your problems will go away. Then you can go back to your mental, physical, environmental, and dietary abuse.

Excuse me, we were talking about Samantha. When her doctor prescribed enalapril after the prednisone, I had to understand what enalapril was all about before I said it was okay for Samantha to take. I'm like that with my doctor: I need to know what you are giving me and what the side effects are. I do not believe in little miracle pills.

We have this high blood pressure drug enalapril. The blood-pressure-lowering effect of enalapril is combined with diuretic drugs and beta-blockers. That can cause a rapid drop in blood pressure. Take it in the morning, and you could pass out on the train, driving, or at school, as in Samantha's case.

Another reason to use this drug with caution is that it's in the class of drugs called angkiotenish-converting-enzyme inhibitors (ACE inhibitors). Enalapril prevents the constriction (narrowing) of blood vessels. In addition, its side effects are chest pain, abdominal pain, cardiac arrest, diarrhea, vomiting, dry mouth, muscle cramps, depression, vertigo, confusion, ataxia, insomnia, nervousness, pneumonia, bronchitis, cough, asthma, upper respiratory infection, exfoliate-dermatitis, toxic epidermal-necrolysis, photosensitivity, blurred vision, renal failure, urinary tract infection, and impotence.

When the doctor prescribed it, I simply thought that it would lower Samantha's blood pressure. Her blood pressure was high in the morning; therefore, I gave her enalapril in the morning. She passed out in school. At that point we had prednisone, enalapril, and all the side effects that the doctors were trying to deal with.

Another doctor prescribed cytoxan. It is one of those immunosuppressive drugs that are an alternative to high doses of corticosteroid (prednisone). Unfortunately, cytoxan may increase a child's risk of developing certain forms of cancer. Moreover, it may interfere with fertility. The less serious side effects include closing of the throat, swelling of the lips and tongue, or a breakout of hives. This drug would be administered through a hole in Samantha's chest. I said no to cytoxan.

Another doctor prescribed plaquenil. Now plaquenil is an antimalarial drug. It is helpful for rheumatic diseases like rheumatoid arthritis and, in this case, lupus. Plaquenil (hydroxychlorguine) is the lesser of the evil drugs. As I said, it can cause retinal toxicity over a long period, but in comparison to some of the other risks, this seemed small. For this reason, I figured we would give Samantha plaquenil to get rid of prednisone. With prednisone gone, Samantha's blood pressure would go to normal, and we get rid of enalapril.

Then another doctor prescribed coumadin, an anticoagulant. It acts by inhabiting vitamin K-dependant coagulant factors. Its side effects are hemorrhages—sometimes fatal ones—from any tissue or organ as well as dizziness and difficulty breathing. Complications may appear as paralysis paresthesia, headaches, or unexplained swelling. Anticoagulant therapy is extremely risky and unstable. I said no to anticoagulant drugs.

Medical Mystery

No one understands what the cause of lupus is. In addition, no one understands how the recommended drugs help lupus patients if they work at all. In any case, a lupus patient may develop a spontaneous blood clot that can lead to a stroke or pulmonary embolism if a clot breaks away and is carried to the heart or lungs, respectively.

A blood clot (platelet aggregation) is when blood forms a small net-like cobweb across a blood vessel, and platelets stick together (aggregate). Natural vitamin E will reduce platelet aggregation. Garlic acts in the same way. Both are more stable and have no side effects.

In retrospect, I find it difficult to believe that I am trying to expatiate a history of all the doctor visits and drugs from seven years to date. In addition to that, I'm trying to understand the doctor of pediatric hematology's frame of reference; his books of diagnosis, treatment, and drugs; the treatment of side effects; and maintaining effective control of the disease and the drugs used for treatment. Next comes the doctor of pediatric nephrology and hypertension, for whom I go through the same list of things to learn. The there's doctor of rheumatology.... One can imagine that it can lead to many drugs. I must be clear in what I say to you, parents and patients. Doctors are the right people, doing the right thing by the book. For your best interests and best health, cooperation is essential.

However, we do not have the science today to understand the human immune system. The chemical and electrical reactions and interactions are incredible and complex. It is a biochemical marvel, the army of cells to protect the body from bacteria, drugs, chemicals, virus, and cancer. It makes you cough and sneeze, create skin secretions and perspiration. It's in everything from lysozyme to lactoperoxidase in mother's milk, to hydrochloric acid. All eject, kill, or inhibit bacteria.

There are normal flora resident bacteria and bacteria that live all over the body. And the immune system is in every part of the body. T cells, B cells, killer T cells, antigen presenting macrophage (APCs), and pattern recognition receptors that are passed from generation to generation. There are the lymph system stem cells in bone marrow, hematopiesis memory cells, helper cells, catatonic cells, suppressor cells, attachment of antigen and cell receptors, self- vs. nonself-recognition, and much more. Clearly, the immune system is there to protect the body even if we cannot understand the complexity of it all.

One would assume in autoimmune diseases that this amazing, unimaginable immune system chemistry breaks down. If your mental frame of reference is the dissection room, and human beings are machines, the parts break down. Then your doctor's assumptions are correct.

In autoimmune diseases, the immune system is doing its job protecting the body. To understand this, one could think of Type 1 diabetes in children who are allergic to cow's milk. The immune system attacks the pancreas because a protein in the pancreas is similar to a protein in cow's milk. With lupus, a person may be allergic to wheat or any one of the chemicals in food, or perhaps environmental free radicals. The immune system is protecting the body by destroying cells of the body because it thinks the cells are invaders.

Modern therapy for lupus is to suppress the immune system. If you must suppress the immune system, then try scorpion venom. It will work better then prednisone.

From the onset of all this, one question in my mind was

what the immune system would do if you lived in outer space and there were no free radicals; no preservatives (such as sodium nitrate, benzoate, sulfites, BHT, and BHA); no salt (which greatly stresses the kidneys' ability to maintain proper fluid volume, causes high blood pressure, and water retention); no refined sugar, corn syrup, or other things harmful to blood sugar control; and no pesticides or herbicides sprayed on or added to crops. These last are some of the worst influences. Over long-term exposure, they can cause cancer and birth defects and in the short-term, vomiting and nerve damage. Forty different pesticides are used on broccoli, one hundred on apples, and fifty on bell peppers. Pesticides penetrate the entire fruit or vegetable and cannot be washed off.

What if there were also no artificial food coloring? FDIC yellow dye # 5 bartizaned, for example, increases the number of mass cells in the body producing histamines. There also wouldn't be any other allergic compounds responsible for allergies, such as asthma, eczema, and hives; carcinogens; or heavy metals, such as lead, mercury, labium, arsenic, nickel, and aluminum solvents. And what if all your body organs—liver, heart, kidneys, and so on—were in perfect health. What would your immune system do? Would you have lupus? Would the immune system be out of a job? Perhaps this mysterious disease is not so mysterious after all. Maybe. But we do not live in outer space. We live in dirty cities with bad chemicals in our food and air.

I asked the doctors what would happen. They said the immune system is still. I was thinking it would do nothing. And at the time, I had a nine-year-old child with a five-year life term with an immune system in her that will eat dirt, viruses, dead particle matter, bacteria, parasites, infections, free radicals, carcinogens, and any organ or cell affected by any or all of this. How to turn this child into a biologically clean healthy human?

The time has come to talk of many things: of treatments, drugs, and doctors; of what to eat and what not to eat; and of what drugs to take and what drugs not to take. Do you want to live to live, or live to die. Look at Samantha and you tell me.

Out with the Garbage

Let us start by eliminating BHT and BHA. BHA and BHT causes cancer in rats. In research with rats, the rats' hair fell out; their blood cholesterol went crazy; and their little baby rats were born with no eyes. Read the food labels, and keep it out of your diet.

Second, do not eat any wheat products. Lupus includes an allergic reaction to wheat and therefore everything that is made with wheat. No food coloring either. It is not going to be easy; however, your life is worth it.

No salt. You do not want your high blood pressure to get higher if you have high blood pressure from your prednisone. You do not want it out of control, and salt will stress out your kidneys, which is the last thing you want. No sodium nitrates. I am talking about most of the cereals you buy in your supermarket and all the cold cuts and frankfurters. No refined sugar—the white sugar you put in your coffee. No hydrogenated oil, preserved with chemicals, poison to animals and humans. Do you really think eating this stuff is going to help your lupus? This stuff gives cancer to normal people!

You're already avoiding wheat, but particularly avoid white bread. It is not good bread even for people not allergic to wheat. They take the bran and the wheat germ out of the bread with high-pressure steel rollers. Then they remove the wheat germ and bran, and you have the endosperm. You turn the wheat flour into white flour, and you have white imitation bread. White bread may also have the chemicals monoglycerine and triglycerides, propylene glycol, diakcetyltrataric acid, propylene glycol, carrageen, rice flour, potato starch, sodium stearoyl-z-lactylate, and calcium sulfate. Some of this stuff, such as carrageen, an extract of Irish moss causes cancer and birth defects. Propylene glycol, which is in your white bread to keep it from discoloring, is better known as antifreeze. This white, so-called enriched, flour is in everything: pies, cookies, donuts, sweet rolls, hamburger and hot dog buns, turnovers, pizza dough, macaroni, waffles, and pancakes. This garbage flour has no nutrition, and all the products that are made with this stuff are more garbage. And remember what your immune system will do. It will attack all this garbage, attack these foreign particles, and engulf them. In your case, this means a lupus flare and kidney failure.

Salt causes damage to the body by causing high blood pressure. This damages your blood vessels and leads to heart attacks, strokes, blindness, and paralysis. So no processed foods. Processed foods are loaded with salt. No fast foods; they are also loaded with salt. You do not want iodine excess goiter—massive enlargement of the thyroid gland from too much salt.

Did you know fluoride is a poison? It is in your toothpaste and your drinking water; do not drink city water from your house, wherever you live. Drink bottled water.

Hazardous, poisonous metal can get into your water through the plumbing in your house, and black plastic pipes can release the metal into your drinking water. Food processors can get metal into food through the refining procedures, thus poisoning products like refined sugar and polished white rice. free radicals that your immune system will attack. Lead is in your drinking water from pipes as well as in cosmetics, glazes on dinner plates, walls, and ceilings. It is also released from the exhaust pipes of a million motor vehicles.

Today's meat is injected with chemicals to fatten livestock. These include hormones, chemicals, preservatives, water solutions—dangerous stuff for a lupus patient. You can eat organically grown meat and chicken without the solution added. Try to eat very little meat. It will be better. You can eat chicken, but do not eat the chicken skin or fat.

They also sell organic hot dogs, which are fine. Any kind of sausage that is not organic is bad for you, and your immune system will punish you for it. Sausage has 90 percent fat and artificial flavoring with lots of salt.

Chewing gum has pork grease in it to give it a better mouth flavoring. No junk food from the nearby burger place. The burger is 75 percent fat, and the cheese is 70 percent fat. Cheap salad dressing has fat in it; even the bun has some fat in it. That is why it tastes so good. French fries are about 60 percent fat and have vegetable oil, refined sugar, and lots of salt.

You do not want to eat pork fat. Margarine is mostly lard, and lard is made from pork fat. About cholesterol, do not take cholesterol drugs. They have many bad side effects. If you are worried about reducing your cholesterol level, buy some lecithin capsules. Lecithin makes cholesterol very easy to dissolve in the blood. Nonprocessed foods have plenty of lecithin. Cholesterol is essential to the human metabolism. Cholesterol is made in the adrenal gland and the liver, and it is vital to survival. If you do not eat it, your body will make it; your body produces it to maintain your daily needs.

Do not drink soda or soft drinks; they are mostly water with refined sugar or a substitute sugar like corn syrup. Cola drinks contain BVD, bromentad, vegetable oil, and corn sesame or cotton seed oil They are doped up with poisonous chemicals. When BVD was given to rats, for instance, they suffered damage to their hearts, livers, thyroid glands, and kidneys. So no soda. No citrus flavored drinks or snack foods, which have many free radicals.

My child is not of drinking age, but you may be. If so, no alcoholic beverages. Why? Because alcoholic beverages are not controlled by the FDA. The internal revenue services are in charge. Ingredients are not put on labels. Beer, for example, has certain artificial coloring, chemicals, EDTA, propyleneglycolalegente, and additives. No one knows about. Wine, has about 70 percent synthetic chemicals in it. Wine can contain copper, sulfate, sulfur dioxide, PVC, or polyvinyl chloride, a chemical that causes liver cancer. Beer has in it diethylpyrocarbonate (DEPC) to kill germs. DEPC is also a cancer producing agent, though. None of this is on the label, and it does not have to be by law. Again, you do not want your immune system to be activated by all this garbage.

Let us go back to being in outer space. What if your immune system had nothing to attack? Would it attack you? So our goal is to clean the body, have strong healthy organs, and not eat garbage food. Our first concern is what we eat as a person living with lupus. You should not eat any of these things I've mentioned. However, who am I to say such things? I started with a nine-year-old child. I could tell her what to eat. I just did not buy the garbage food at the supermarket. You, Miss Know-it-all? Have your beer, pizza, your MacDonald's, all your snacks, and feel very good. Then comes the day, and it will come, that you are lying in the hospital with all those tubes hanging out of your body. And you say, "Oh God, what are you doing to me, doctor?" What you should be saying is, "Oh God, what did I do to myself?" And the hospital gives you more of that garbage food that gives you lupus. Your immune system eats the garbage and more of you, and you say, "Doctor, give me that miracle pill and save me so I can go home and eat Mac D's and smoke a blunt and drink beer and feel very good."

Then you lose your kidney. And you say, "Oh God, what are you doing to me doctor? Give me that miracle pill, and all this will go away." And one day you go to happy land.

Do you want to take the journey with me and live? Or do you want to go to happy land, Miss Know-it-all? It is your call. Let me repeat myself: my daughter was nine years old when she was diagnosed with lupus. You may not be nine years old; you may be the one person who knows everything about lupus. Who can tell you anything? You have all the lupus problems and you may die. Why is Samantha living as a normal teenager with no lupus problems? I can tell you that Samantha is in remission.

My friend, you are a very special person with a life-threatening disease called lupus. I can never understand your mental frame of reference, and you can never understand my mental frame of reference because we are not each other. Yet I can tell you what I was thinking six years ago when Samantha was diagnosed with lupus. I was thinking that if I could get the immune system to sit around and do nothing, then nothing would happen. The premise that one could live in outer space is a good one. It may just eliminate the allergy that's causing your lupus. I can tell you how to live with such a premise. However, as they say, you can lead a horse to the water but you cannot make him drink. Okay, you are not a horse, but I will try to lead, nonetheless.

Creating a clean body internally and strengthening all the major organs is what we are trying to do. In the process, you just may eliminate the cause of your lupus. Let us eliminate the bad stuff. No wheat. No salt. (That is almost impossible today, but go for low salt or no salt foods.) No refined sugar or any of its forms (corn syrup, etc.). No junk food, no alcohol, no pot, or weed, no drugs of any kind except what your doctor gives you. Eat organic foods, which are foods with no carcinogenic chemicals. If you do not have the money to buy all organic foods, then buy only American-grown fruits and vegetables. Peel all the fruits. If it does not have a peel, then wash all vegetables. They sell a veggie wash; buy it and use it to clean your vegetables. Eat raw green peppers and carrots every day as well as lettuce and tomatoes when you can.

Once a month you can eat organic meat. Never eat pork. You can eat lots of chicken if it has no preservatives, hormones, or solutions added. Do not eat the chicken skin. Use olive oil to cook with, not margarine. Use real butter, garlic, onions, and in the morning eat organic cereal made from brown rice with organic nonfat milk, or 1 percent milk.
Restaurants are dirty. Only God knows were they are getting their food from. If you must eat out, choose chicken teriyaki at the sushi place or chicken broccoli from a Chinese restaurant that doesn't use MSG. You can also try chicken and black beans from the Mexican place, but that's it for restaurant food.

Hey, you can eat whatever you want. I am telling you what we do. If you cannot afford organic meat and frankfurters, do not eat them at all.

Some days it is smart not to eat solid food for a day or two. Drink lots of spring water and organic juices. You can make homemade juices: just get some apples, oranges, or whatever you like, and blend them in a blender with some spring water. And for one day now and then, just drink juices. If you must eat, try eating natural snacks like peanuts, fruits, and raisins. Carry your natural snacks around with you. When your friends eat all that garbage, you eat your natural snacks—organic if you can get them.

Sodium nitrate should especially be avoided. It is a preservative that, once in the stomach, can combine with substances known as secondary amino to create new compounds known as nitro amines. That is a powerful cancer-causing chemical, and your immune system will react to all of this. You need to avoid free radical lipid per oxidation. We are trying not to activate the immune system. Therefore, if you can stop eating garbage food, then you can move on to the next thing you must do to live in good health with no pain and no death sentence.

The next thing to do is to reinforce and strengthen every organ in the body. We'll focus on the major organs, the heart, liver, and kidneys. To accomplish this, you take a powerful antioxidant, a nutrient called ubiquinone, or coenzyme Q10, which helps the metabolic reaction of transforming food into energy in the mitochondria—the area of the cells that produce energy. The heart and liver need a lot of energy. CoQ10 exists in the membranes of the mitochondria, which are responsible for generating 95 percent of the total energy needed by the human body. It performs its critical function, the manufacture of adenosine troposphere (ATP), the basic energy molecule of the cell. There are high concentrations of CoQ10 in the organs that need the largest supplies of energy, including the heart and the liver, although CoQ10 plays a vital role in all organs of the body. Studies have shown that if the essential levels of CoQ10 are allowed to decline, the results are poor health and disease.

CoQ10 has also been found to act as an antioxidant and protects cells from free radicals. Free radicals are highly charged ions that damage cell membranes. Pathologic effects are cancer and atherosclerosis through lipid peroxides. CoQ10 is one of the lipid peroxide inhibitors. Another good aspect of CoQ10 is that it will lower your blood pressure, and it works well for periodontal health. It is well known for strengthening the heart from a cellular level. Toxicological testing of human subjects has shown no risk of toxicity from CoQ10.

All right, so far we have eliminated almost all the food in your supermarket—all that processed garbage, all that chemical poison, BHT, and cancer causing sodium nitrate in your cold cuts. Come on, you do not want to eat all that stuff. Then why is it there, you ask? In my next book, I will explain why. What is important is not eating all that bad food. You're now taking 60mg of CoQ10 each day. Buy it on sale at the big super centers. Buy name brands like Nature's Bounty. The store brands cost less; however, they are not what they claim. No one regulates herbs and vitamins; therefore, they do not have to put the right stuff in the product. And most of the time, it is not in there. You need good antioxidants. What you eat is important because your immune system is going to react to dirty or bad food or chemicals that should not be in your body, and your immune system reacting to invaders kills both the invaders and the cells that are affected.

More on Free Radicals

There are environmental sources of free radicals, such as oxidizing agents. Included are ionizing radiation from industry sun exposure; cosmic rays; medical X-rays; ozone; nitrous oxide; automobile exhaust; heavy metals, such as mercury, cadmium, and lead; cigarette smoke, both active and passive; and alcohol.

Unsaturated fat may create a strain on the natural antioxidants of the body. Other chemicals and compounds from food, water, and air also strain the organs when these free radicals enter the body and interact with healthy tissue, setting off potentially damaging reactions. Free radicals are believed to play a role in more than sixty different health conditions including the ageing process itself, cancer, and arteriosclerosis. Reducing exposure to free radicals and increasing your intake of antioxidants and nutrients can reduce the risk of free radical related health problems. Free radicals are inherently unstable because they contain extra energy. To reduce their energy load, free radicals react with certain cells in the body, thus interfering with the cells' ability to function normally. Fortunately, many natural antioxidants interfere with free radicals before they can damage the body.

Antioxidants work in several ways. They may reduce the energy of free radicals or stop the free radical from forming in the first place. Or they may interrupt an oxidizing chain reaction to minimize the damage of free radicals. Superoxide dismutase (SOD), catalase, and glutathione peroxide are enzymes produced by the body itself to defuse many types of free radicals. Supplements of these compounds are also available to augment the body's supply. Selenium enhances the antioxidant effects of

Vitamin E. In addition, vitamins and many enzymes and minerals act as antioxidants. The best way to provide the body with complete protection against free radical damage is through supplements.

Vitamin E has been found to reduce the damage to chromosomes and DNA by carcinogens. It also reduces the incidents of cancer in laboratory animals fed carcinogens by interfering with harmful free radical reactions. It acts to block the oxidation that can turn lipids into harmful peroxide. Vitamin E could be called a free radical scavenger. It minimizes the damage done by being a free radical chain breaker. Free radical reactions can never be stopped entirely, but vitamin E and other antioxidants can significantly reduce the rate at which they occur. You need to take 800 IU of natural vitamin E (d-alpha tocopheryl) per day.

The cell membranes are of critical importance in the health and longevity of cells because it's the membranes that actively transport all the vitamins minerals, trace metals, nutrients, and hormones. Therefore, maintaining healthy function in these membranes can be considered one of the most important aspects of health at the biochemical level. The cell membrane is a kind of sandwich, or bi-layer, of fat-like molecules with cholesterol between them and selected proteins trapped in this system. Vitamin E sits in the very middle of this fatty bi-layer and protects the fats from reacting with oxygen in a manner that damages the cell—oxidative damage. This damage can be caused by chemicals in the environment, such as ozone in smog. Vitamin E serves as a powerful sink, trapping oxidants that chemically alter membrane components and weaken the membrane, and thus, the entire cell. A weakened membrane means weaker resistance to diseases.

Vitamin E also reduces the danger of blood clots, heart attacks, strokes, and pulmonary embolism (when a clot breaks away and is carried to the lungs). All of these related problems arise when blood platelets attach themselves and stick together (aggregate) in a clump, attracting long strands of fiber in the blood vessels. When laboratory rats were fed vitamin E, blood platelet aggregation was remarkably reduced, even dropping to normal range. Similar effects appear to occur in humans who take vitamin E supplements.

The effects of vitamin E on platelet aggregation and platelet count are involved in the origin of vascular pathology. Researchers reported that platelet counts were reduced in about one third of a group of adults consuming between 100 IU and 800 IU of vitamin E daily. Long-term supplementation with vitamin E, approximately 800 IU per day, prolonged blood clotting time. Vitamin E is a major biologic oxidative agent and a natural defense against poisonous gas for people who live in larger cities with automotive and industrial pollution and the crippling effect of phagocytes, free radicals, and lipid peroxides. These things are associated with cancer. Phagocytes are a result of the formation of free radicals and lipid peroxides, two substances that are highly unstable chemicals created by the unusual oxidizing power of ozone. Doctors observed that animals exposed to ozone without the protection of vitamin E suffered hemolytic (destruction of red blood cells) at the rate of 80 percent or more. The animals fed vitamin E. suffered a lesser rate of hemolytic pollution.

Sources of ozone are any equipment around the house that produces sparks or static discharge, as well as ultraviolet or other ionizing radiation. Also, units may be in operation in offices and elevators that produce ozone. Some products of distilled water have ozone as well. Companies actually add this poisonous gas to their product without regard as to whether it is used for baby formula. The relationship between distilled water and crib deaths should be investigated. However, that is another book.

Free radicals are capable of destroying an enzyme or protein or DNA that fuse together. Then havoc occurs when the normally orderly arrangement of enzymes and other components are disturbed. Damage from free radicals can occur in different ways, such as cross–linking, in which free radical reaction cause proteins and/or DNA to fuse together. This causes molecule damage and membrane damage, allowing free radical reactions to destroy the integrity of the cell. Membranes then interfere with the cell's ability to bring nutrients and expel wastes. Another method is lipid per oxidation, which causes fat compounds in the body to turn rancid. Age pigments interfere with cell chemistry and rupture lysosome membranes. Hydrolyze destroys cellular tissue, also rupturing the cell membranes. Clearly, we need to detoxify all pollutants. Even daily exposure to background radiation produces enough damage to cause cancer.

Selenium, like CoQ10, is an antioxidant. It can detoxify heavy metals, protect against environmental carcinogens, stabilize blood pressure, and stimulate the immune system in a good way. It can prevent cancer and monoclonal proliferation by improving the health of muscle cells. It also promotes CoQ10 in the heart muscle cells, which, as we said, is vital energy for healthy functions.

Selenium works with vitamin E as a powerful antioxidant to activate needed thyroid hormones that are proven to protect against free radicals and cell damage. Selenium and vitamin E bind to pollutants to prevent their absorption. They increase the excretion of arsenic into bile and alter the tissue disposition of lead, mercury, cadmium, silver, and thallium, an overall protective effect. This is especially important because lead pollution from burning gasoline causes brain damage. Mercury, a well-known potential poison, comes from industry pesticides. Cadmium pollution from cigarettes causes high blood pressure. Vitamin E and selenium together can protect you.

Think about all the garbage out there. As much as you can, you need to stop eating, drinking, breathing free radicals, whether it's pot, cigarette smoke, industrial waste, tap water, mercury-poisoned fish, or anything else. (Interestingly enough, tuna containing mercury is less dangerous than other sources because selenium concentrates in tuna, reduces the toxicity of the ingested mercury.) You need to understand what you eat, the drugs your doctor gives you, the air you are breathing. It is essential to good health. If you do not take the time to understand, only God can help you, my friend. And you can talk to him about it when you get to happy land. Fortunately most of the environmental toxins that cause disease can be eliminated or neutralized in the body by taking high doses of antioxidants.

Vitamin C is one thing you need in high doses. I am talking about 1,000 to 10,000 mg per day. And even 10,000 mg to 20,000 mg per day, if you can manage it. High doses of vitamin C will deplete copper in the body, though, so supplement with copper—3 mg of copper per day.

Most mammals produce ascorbic acid (vitamin C) in their bodies, saturating blood and tissue. Humans today do not, although our primate ancestors produced it in the liver as an enzyme, L-gulonolactone oxidase, for ascorbic acid synthesis. Somehow it got lost in our evolution, and it is amazing that we have survived the vitamin C deficiency. Scurvy, for example, is a disorder from lack of vitamin C. Other problems due to deficiency include infectious diseases, low back pain, arthritis, inflammation, defective wound healing, bleeding gums, defective collagen, defective metabolism, and lack of connective tissue.

Everyone knows vitamin C will help you get rid of that cold or flu and prevent you from getting another. Vitamin C is a lot more than that. It will help phagocytes (white blood cells) that kill bacteria and viruses. Vitamin C is an antibiotic in and of itself. It will increase your resistance to cancer by strengthening the natural defenses against environmental toxins. The phagocytes require a lot of vitamin C, and the recommended daily doses are insignificant for good health in humans. So what is a good intake of vitamin C?

To maintain good health, first let me say that there is a complete lack of toxicity in high doses of ascorbic acid. The more you take, the healthier you become. A gorilla consumes about 5 grams of vitamin C per day from his diet of vegetation. Everyone's needs are different. You can take 1,000 mg a week and add 1,000 mg every week until your stools soften. Then, back down 1,000 mg and stay with what you have. That is the amount your body needs be, whether it's 1,000mg a week or 20,000 mg a week. If you can manage it, 20,000 mg a week is better.

You especially need lots of vitamin C when under stress, and lupus can cause a lot of stress. For your health, try to also minimize the stress with herbs. Whenever Samantha is stressed for any reason, I give her valerian root. Valerian root has been around for centuries and was used by the Greek physician Dioscorides for liver problems, insomnia, and sedation of the central nervous system. Stress is a major cause of disease and damage, so stay on top of it.

Milk thistle is a plant found in Western Europe and in some parts of the United States. The leaves and seeds are used for stomach problems. The seeds are good for the liver and kidneys because they contain a bioflavoid known as silymarin, which works by blocking the entrance of harmful toxins and removing toxins from cells. It can also regenerate injured liver cells.

Green tea extract is also beneficial. Samantha will not drink green tea, so I give her green tea extract. One should drink four cups of green tea per day. Green tea contains caffeine so you don't want to drink so much that you get the caffeine-related problems, such as insomnia, anxiety, and sleep deprivation, which can lead to a host of diseases. Green tea contains polyphenols catechin called epigallocatechin gallate (EGCG), which promotes good health. It prevents cardiovascular disease, lowers cholesterol levels, stimulates the immune system cells, is antibacterial, relieves aches and pains, soothes depression, and aids digestion. In short, it's a good tea to drink.

The body also needs folic acid for DNA synthesis and to keep amino acids from rising in the blood and causing strokes. If you live in a western society, you are folic acid deficient. Deficiency can cause cardiovascular disease and eventually death, so finding a good folic acid supplement is essential.

Garlic stimulates digestion, lowers blood pressure, and helps prevent arteriosclerosis. If you do not like the taste of garlic, you can find supplements for that as well.

There are more supplements you need, and I will give you a list of all that Samantha has been taking and is taking today.

Conclusion

In the final analysis, we get to the good part. I do not mean drinking beer, getting stoned, smoking a blunt, and eating Mac D's. You will go to happy land with all those tubes hanging out of your body if you do not get it together, trust me girl. Here again is the food Samantha will not eat.

No wheat or anything made with wheat. No white bread. White bread has no value. It is made with overrefined flour and pumped up with air and preservatives. Do not eat it. No preservatives, no salt. There is no salt in our house, and we try to keep it out of our food. Salt is in almost everything you buy today. Therefore, we buy low-salt or no-salt products. No BHT, BHA, or any chemical names you do not understand. Fruits and vegetables have tons of pesticides, so wash your fruits and vegetables. It's best to buy organic. No sodium nitrates, which are in all cold cuts. They will make you sick and give you cancer. No refined sugar (white sugar) corn syrup, or ice cream. (You can eat frozen yogurt instead.) Do not eat junk food. You do not want lupus flare-ups, and the chemical hydrolyzing can give you lupus flare-ups. It is in FD&C yellow #5, cosmetics, food, pesticides, and dyes. No mushrooms or soft drinks. There are bad chemicals in beef, pork, lamb, and veal. The chemicals are there to fatten the livestock.

If you went to one of the factories that processed food, you would never eat that stuff again. Let's face it: one can never stop rats, insects, and bacteria. You can try using lots of chemicals; you can even put the chemicals in the food (scary, but true), but you can't eliminate them. Eat fresh organic, natural, no preservative food. Again, do not eat chemicals you cannot identify.

Samantha eats lots of natural preservative-free chicken breast and drumsticks, along with organic green peppers, potatoes, and lettuces. I cook everything in olive oil. As for natural products, be careful. They may say natural and still have preservatives and chemicals and sugar and salt. If they do, do not eat them.

If your doctor has you on prednisone, ask your doctor to put you on plaquenil. Yes, the doctor knows best, and you are the patient. Still, your relationship with your doctor must be one of mutual cooperation. You must understand your disease, the treatments for your disease, and the idea that you need an alternative to prednisone. You need a less dangerous drug. The goal is to get off prednisone as we strengthen all the major organs and add long-term supplements of antioxidants to clean the body of free radical damage. That may well be the cause of lupus.

Taking antimalarial drugs can cause vision problems from deposits of the drug in the cornea and more serious problems to the retina, which can cause total blindness. Again, the safe dosage is 200 mg every other day, not the recommended 200 mg every day. To help prevent damage to the eyes, Samantha takes bilberry extract. It is used to improve vision, does not interact with commonly prescribed drugs, and has no side effects. Also lutein, an antioxidant, protects the retina of the eye from macular degeneration and has no side effects.

Here is the list of nutrients, supplements, and herbs that Samantha has been taking every day for the past six years.

CoQ10 (60 mg per day)

Natural vitamin E d-alpha tocopherol (800 IU per day)

- Selenium (200 mg per day)

- Milk thistle (175 mg per day)

- Green tea extract (300 mg per day)

- Folic acid (400 mcg per day)

- Vitamin C (500 mg per day)

- Garlic capsules (1000 mg per day)

- Bilberry extracts (125 mg per day)

- Astragals (1,500 mg per day)

- Grape seed extract (150 mg per day)

- Omega-3 fish oil (1000 mg per day)

Flaxseed oil if you don't like the fish taste (fish oil is better)

- Glucosamine sulfate (500 mg per day)

- Calcium plus vitamin D (600 mg per day)

- Vitamin B 6 (100 mg per day)

- Lutein (20 mg per day)

You are thinking, "If I take all this stuff, will it work for me?" Well, I have had control of Samantha's diet and have given her all this stuff, and it works for her. Samantha's condition is in remission. You may experience a dramatic improvement in your condition and enjoy many years of good health. I can only tell you of Samantha's life. You determine your life.

Let's quickly go over the nutritional supplements and herbs and what they do for you.

Vitamin C: prevents colds, allergies, backaches, atherosclerosis, cataracts, diabetes, glaucoma, high cholesterol, high blood pressure, and many more diseases
Side effects: extremely safe, some people get diarrhea at high doses.

Glucosamine sulfate: helps prevent kidney stones and osteoarthritis
Side effects: Some glucosamine may be processed with salt, a problem for people with high blood pressure.

Grapeseed extract: prevents varicose veins and heart attacks
Side effects: no known side effects

Calcium plus vitamin D: prevents fractures, promotes healthy teeth and bones, beneficial to blood pressure and nerve cells, and prevents osteoarthritis and rickets
Side effects: People with kidney problems should not take calcium.

CoQ10: crucial to cell energy, protects the body from heart

attacks, periodontal support, stimulates the immune system, counters histamine effects, acts as antioxidant
Side effects: no known side effects, extremely safe

Bilberry extract: acts as antioxidant, supports connective tissue, and helps retinopathy, circulation, and macular degeneration

Flaxseed oil: anti-inflammatory, no fish smell, may not work as well as fish oil because it may not lower triglyceride to protect the heart
Side effects: no known side effects.

Garlic: stimulates digestive organs, acts as antibacterial action, and reduces clotting
Side effect: no known side effects

Selenium: activates the antioxidant glutathione peroxide, which can prevent some diseases, such as cancer and rheumatoid arthritis; improves energy; protects cell membranes; helps produce CoQ10 and prostaglandins in the body; neutralizes cadmium; and detoxifies free radicals
Side effects: You may get a skin rash if you take 1000 mg or more per day.

Milk thistle: supports the liver, regenerates liver tissue, lowers cholesterol, and acts as an antidote to poison mushrooms
Side effects: no known side effects

Green tea: prevents cancer, promotes weight loss, acts as an antioxidant, treats atherosclerosis, and neutralizes free radicals
Side effects: no known side effects.

Astragals: supports immune system
Side effects: no known side effects.

Omega-3 fish oil: acts as an anti-inflammatory and prevents
diabetes, high blood pressure, and rheumatoid arthritis
Side effects: Some people have gastrointestinal upset.

Vitamin B6: supports neurotransmitter substances, prevents
heart disease, and is a treatment for carpal tunnel syndrome
Side effects: Large doses over 2000 mg per day can cause nerve
damage.

Natural vitamin E (d-alpha tocopherol): protects cell
membranes, fights ozone damage, and reduces the risk of heart
disease, cataracts, high cholesterol, osteoarthritis, and blood
clots
Side effects: no known side effects

Folic acid: synthesizes DNA and prevents heart disease. Folic
acid deficiency can lead to depression, high cholesterol,
osteoporosis, and birth defects.

Though this may seem like a lot, keep in mind that Samantha
takes no prescription drugs and is in remission. So there you
have it, I have just spilt my guts talking to myself. I remember
the frustration, pain, fear, and prayers after the diagnosis. I
understand spontaneous remissions.

And by God, the day is ours. This book is not a cure for lupus; it
is an account of a child who is a teenager today who has lupus

yet lives a healthy life. She has no lupus-related problems. It may be one thing or a combination of all the things we do that stabilizes her condition. In the final analysis, though, it is working, and we continue to move in the same direction with the help of God, family, and friends.

Acknowledgments

Special thanks to the doctors who helped me understand a mysterious disease. There have been times when we disagreed, but they have always been good friends, for today and tomorrow.

Dr. Steven David Styler
Dr. Juan C. Kupferman
Dr. Shipar Kaicke
Dr. Laura Barenstein
Dr. Norman Saffra
Dr. Kathleen M. O'Day